Maca Root: An Up And Coming Nutrient That Improves Sexual Performance And Fertility

Disclaimer and Terms of Use: Effort has been made to ensure that the information in this book is accurate and complete, however, the author and the publisher do not warrant the accuracy of the information, text and graphics contained within the book due to the rapidly changing nature of science, research, known and unknown facts and internet. The Author and the publisher do not hold any responsibility for errors, omissions or contrary interpretation of the subject matter herein. This book is presented solely for motivational and informational purposes only.

Table of Contents

Introduction

People who are addicted to coffee or tea in their morning to get boosted should know about maca root. Its root resembles potato and it has stimulating effect on brain just like tea of coffee that gives you fresh start to your day. The only positive side is being that unlike coffee, it doesn't contain caffeine which serves as a health factor to your body. It is also being popular as an energy booster after heavy workout or morning jogging. It charges up your activity by supplying nutritional vitamins and minerals. Maca root is herbal plant that is in the trend as beneficial in improving sexual performance. Medical research has also claimed to be effective among fertility affected people. In Spanish it is popular as maca-maca. Maca root is not a newly discovered root plant; in 1843 it was first brought into notice by Gerhard Walpers.

Maca root is found commonly in mountains of Peru. Although it is used for medicinal purpose, Maca was also cultivated as a crop for home use. It has aroma that is similar to butterscotch. Maca can is eaten in many forms.

Nutritional Information

Maca serves great nutritional value and it is one of the rich sources of minerals. It also contains amino acids, energy vitamins (B-12) and enzymes. It has significant value in remineralization of body. Maca assists in maintaining hormonal balance in the system and keeps hormonal fluctuation under control.

Common Usage

- In many baked preparations and in roasted items

- In many health and fermented drinks like maca chia.

- It is used as a powder form to top up in vegetable salad preparation or also can be used to make soup.

- In farms it also being used to make land more fertile to get more quality crops

Clinical Usage

Apart from its importance in increasing sexual desire and fertility, it serves many more medicinal purposes as follows

- Used in the treatment of anemia, also called as "tired blood" and also in chronic fatigue syndrome.

- For increasing stamina and energy level in the body.

- Used my athletes to increased performance and endurance level.

- As a memory enhancer

- For women it has role in improving hormonal imbalance, menstrual bleeding problems and in early menopause cases.

- Other usage includes treatment of weak bones, cancer of stomach, erectile dysfunction etc.

Side Effects

Studies have shown little side effects of Maca in the regular users who consume it less than 3 grams every day. Average consumers have shown good tolerance capacity to maca. Although due to absence of valid information on use of maca during pregnancy, it is advised to avoid using it. According to Health experts it is considered to be safe in consumption based on the data available.

Maca As A Natural Libido Booster

In recent few times, Maca has generated a great buzz due to its role in generating more libidos. It is also mentioned in ancient culture of Incan about its effect in increasing sexuality level. This legendary plant is famous for sexuality enhancer for more than two thousand years.

This herbal plant has a chain of information passed on from generations to generations on its performance check on sexuality and fertility. Although there is little evidences found in the support of its medicinal and sexual effect theories.

Research or studies conclusion

Some randomized researches were carried out that showed beneficial effect in improving fertility among men. These researches have claimed that maca roots has been effective in

- Improving quality and quantity of semen.

- Treatment of early menopause symptoms

- Enlarged prostate making it less in size over some procedure time.

Animal Studies

Maca studies have been also carried out on animals but not humans. Human studies are lacking in many numbers compared to the ones on animals. The results are more or less the same on positive side to increase sexuality performances.

These animal studies have been carried out suggests that it is aphrodisiac in nature; aphrodisiac means any substance that improve sexual performances desire. Even though there are little evidences maca in effective or note, many doctors have said that have seen the sperm count goes high as compared to few days.

Types Of Maca Root Powder And Its Various Health Benefits

Due its plethora of flooding health benefits to people, maca root are being considered to be in the category of super food item. Most People know maca root as general, but few knows that there are many forms of maca roots being cultivated and many forms of maca roots are available to consumption for home and commercial usage. These forms have different effects on different parts of body organs.

There Are Primarily Three Types Of Maca Roots

- Red Maca root

- Yellow Maca root

- Black Maca root

There Are Basically 3 Form Of Intake Of Maca:

1. **Natural As A Vegetable Root**: They can be eaten as a natural plant.

2. **Tablets:** The roots of the maca are cut and are processed into tablets form so that they can be gulped down along with water easily.

3. **Powder:** The other form of maca root is in powder form which can be taken directly with water or can be sprinkled in any vegetable or fruit and can be had like that.

Red Maca

Red maca powder is considers to be the rare type and it comes under highly popular root. It has almost similar benefits that yellow or brown types of root provide. Red form of maca powder has its own unique taste. Red maca root resembles purple cabbage and beet. It contains high level of antioxidants in it. One big difference between red maca and black maca is that they do not increase the direct volume of the male sperm; this benefit is typical to black maca only. The intake of red maca is very easy and it can be taken in powder form or can be consumed as a direct vegetable root as the taste of the root is very tasty and does not have a bad odor.

Black Maca

Black maca is referred to as a scarlet or even lavender group of maca. They belong to reddish family and it is dark red almost black in color. Black maca is supposed to be different from other two and have very specific benefits. They are supposed to be most beneficial for the latent memory increase and also they are the only maca which is supposed to increase the volume content of the sperm in the male. Along with the increase in the volume of male they also increase the mobility of the sperm. This means that the hitting of the sperm into the fertility organ of female, becomes more and thus the conceiving process is helped greatly with the help of black maca. The fatigue level is also increased in a person who takes black maca in comparison with the other color maca roots. The fatigue time increases to as much as 100 minutes where it originally was just 15 minutes, inside the water body.

Yellow Maca

This is one more kind of maca and also belongs to same family and also has same properties as compared with other two. The main benefit of yellow maca is that it stimulates the fertility process greatly into the male and female.

1. Providing Energy

In the morning time people across globe have a habit of taking tea or coffee so that their day goes on smoothly and they do not feel sleepy. Instead of that, if someone shifts his energy in taking maca roots then it will be really helpful and will definitely boost up the energy level of the person. He need not start his day with the caffeine intake rather start the day with the natural source that provides energy, to continue the day, without many side effects.

2. Maintains The Sexual System Of The Body

The presence of estrogen into our body that comes naturally by its own process, misbalances the other hormonal system of the body. Maca roots stimulate the hypothalamus and also it nourishes the glands like pituitary glands. These glands are the main regulatory glands of our body. They regulate all kinds of hormones in the body. Due to maca, these main glands are regulated and because of this they bring in balance to our other glands like thyroid, pancreas and adrenal glands. Hormones like thyroxin etc are the main source for maintaining the digestive system of our body.

3. Works According To Body

Maca works according to the needs of the body. It does not work individually but rather it adapts to the body condition and then it works in accordance to the body system. If in a body, there is production of too much of a kind of hormone then maca regulars the production and dampens the same and if in some other body there is a lack of some kind of hormone then it regulates that gland helps in proper secretion of that particular hormone. In short, it works differently in different bodies and the way that is best for the body.

4. During Menopause

Maca regulates all kind of gland into our body. They are also helpful for women when they are undergoing the process of menstrual cycle and it also increases the time of start of menopause, which maintains a lot of hormonal balance in women. Menopause is one state after which, the women body undergoes a lot of changes and the women has to bear a lot of frequent mood swings. Menopause brings in some difficulties in the female body and it affects the mental process of the female segment, greatly. Maca helps in delay of the time and thus maintains the female body in correct shape for longer duration.

5. Maca Helps In Relieving Cancer And Depression

Macca regulates the hormones and tissues of the body. Cancer is development of extra unwanted tissue into the body. Now, when maca regulates the tissue of the body it does not allow deposition of any unwanted tissue into the body and thus helps in overcoming any cancer into the body. The root is also a great mood regulator. It helps in maintain a good mood rather a positive mood of the person and thus it keeps depression away from the mind of the person. Depression is nothing but the mental state wherein the person goes into an all time low mood swing and sometimes also leads to suicide attempts on the part of the person. Maca helps in getting over all such mental conditions of the person.

6. Maca Being Nutrient Rich Substance

Maca is one natural substance which has natural enzymes, vitamins and minerals that helps in the regulation of all the other glands and hormones. This is the reason that they can overcome serious disease like depression and cancer. This is the reason that the menopause in the women body is delayed because maca contains such substance that enhances sexual stimulating hormones like estrogen, responsible for smooth menstrual cycle. This menstrual cycle delays the menopause.

7. Easy Consumption

The duration for which the root has to be consumed is very easy. One has to start with a half spoon of the powder and then it can be increased to 2-3 spoons, taken on a daily basis. This increase can be done with in a period of two to three weeks. It is best to keep one day off if the person is taking a dose of three spoons of Maca on a daily basis. The root is easily consumable and one need not keep a lot of safety measure while taking it just that the substance is supposed to be taken at exact time in all the days. The gap of 24 hours should be maintained while taking the dose daily.

8. Easy Medium Of Consumption

One can take half a spoon of maca in any form and there are no hassles in taking the same as the taste of the substance is good and can be consumes easily. One can sprinkle it on top of any fruits like banana. It can be mixed in the soup that one takes.

Salt along with maca root powder is a great way to health and has a perfect delicious taste. It can be taken as a desert as a mixture with honey and maple syrup. It can be mixed in any herbal tea and start a great day with it and it can also be used to sprinkle as a spice in some snacks items like popcorn and any rolls.

9. Good Source Of Pure Protein

Maca contains around 20 % of pure proteins in one ounce of the powder. This is a great way of increasing the proteins in the body and is comparable to the protein content in some plant seed. Proteins are the building blocks of the muscle into our body and it is a must for anyone undergoing the process of heavy workout. After work out is the time when one should take maca because that is the time when the muscle has undergone lot of pressure and is worn down. One will need maca during that time so that it can directly enter the muscles of the body and helps in its recovery and its development.

10.   High Iodine Content

Iodine is supposed to be present in the sea food in high amount and that is the reason that the people taking in high amount of sea food never have to suffer the problems related to thyroid glands. However, for vegetarians who do not take sea food, iodine goes lacking into their body. The plants roots also contain iodine but again these days because of hybrid plants and soil erosion, iodine intake from the body is decreasing. This is the reason that more vegetarians suffer with the problem of thyroid. Now, maca is the perfect source of iodine for the vegetarian mass and they can take the dose of maca and increase the iodine content into their body. Around 20 grams of maca contains 100 micrograms of iodine and one needs around 150 micrograms of iodine into body on a daily basis. If a person is taking maca on a daily basis they do not have to bother about the thyroid gland of their body.

11. Cholesterol Regulator

There are two kind of cholesterol present into our body; good cholesterol and bad cholesterol. The good cholesterol is an important constituent of the body and it should be present in the body in adequate amount so that the bad cholesterol of the body can be eliminated out easily. Bad cholesterol is bad for one's body and should be eliminated out form the body otherwise they will be deposited in muscle and make it fat unnecessarily. Maca is one plant that contains a lot of plant sterols like sitosterol and such and they are the molecules that are most resembling nutrient to good cholesterol and thus can help in reduction of bad cholesterol from the body. Maca roots thus can help our body in overcoming any disease that is related to the heart, by elimination of bad cholesterol which affects the heart the most.

12. Removal Of Food Craving

Maca roots contain almost about 9% of fibers into one ounce of powder. This is a good constituent of fiber a kind of food can have. They help in a lot of ways. Fiber is the material that helps in storage and retention of water into the body for longer duration of time. If one has fibers substance just before lunch and dinner then the consumption of food becomes less in that meal and one eats less of carbohydrates and fats. This helps in maintain the fat content of the body and the person does not become fat. Fiber is also important for the body because they helps in the times of constipation and maintains a proper digestion system into our body. If one has maca powder, sprinkle on the raw vegetable and then have them, it becomes a double benefit for the taker and then it adds on to the fibers content of the salad. This helps in regulation of body process greatly.

13.   Reduce Prostate Enlaggement

Prostate enlargement leads to prostate cancer in the human body and this can be reduced by the intake of Maca root specifically red maca root. This root is very red in color and is very thick in nature. The sexual hormone that is enhanced with the intake of Maca roots, it also stimulates the prostate glands and thus help in stopping prostate cancer into the body. When the sexual hormone is taken along with the testosterone into the body is helps greatly and it chows results within 21 days of the treatment process. The weight of other body parts was not affected during the treatment process, which means that there are no side effects caused by the whole process of the reduction of prostate enlargement.

14.   Increase In Sperm Count

One type of maca root is black maca. This kind of root, epically the fragments of the black roots, is supposed to be effective for the sperm creation of into the body. The fragments of black maca is supposed to contain a substance known as ethyl acetate, which when mixed with one more substance, then it shows a great increase in the sperm level of a person. Males who eat maca can show a great development of the sexual hormone into them because of which the sperm count of the male is increased. This root can also help the male who do not have enough sperm count so that they can help their partner in fertility process. The male can take the black maca fragments in many ways like they can consume it raw and also can make it in a powder form and can take a plain dose of the powder along with water. Maca taken in any way shows a great result into the body of the person and helps his sexual hormones greatly. Apart from being a great help for males it also is a great help for the women segment of society. In female body it helps in the maturation of the egg follicles. This process helps in conceiving of the baby and removes any complication, from the male side and the female side.

15.   Post Menstrual Sexual Activity

After the menopause the sexual activity with the female segment of society deceases greatly and their body is no more into the condition of that process because of non availability of sexual hormone into the female body. This is the main reason for any kind of depression and physical train that the women have to undergo. The anxiety level of the female segment increases because of this and they remain in a constant state of depression after menopause hit their body. This is the time when maca roots comes in handy and they stimulate the growth of sexual desire into the body of female and thus maintains the anxiety and depression level of the female. A normal dosage of around 5 grams is enough, on a daily basis, to maintain the proper body functions of the female segment of society. This process does not change the other hormone level of the body thus causing no harm and side effects into the female body.

16.   Sexual Hormone Affecting Female Bones

Once the female body has reached menopause and the secretion of sexual glands slows down, then it also affects the bone structure of the body and the strength of the bones is decreased into the body. In some cases it also affects the height of the female. This entire sexual hormonal related problem can be resolved with the intake of maca roots as they are supposed to increase the sexual hormone inside the human body. They also contain some amount of calcium into them which affects the bone structure of the body positively and thus helps in proper maintenance of bones in the older age. The bone mineral density which is lost due to the loss of estrogen, the sexual hormone of the female body, is regained again with the usage of maca roots by the women past age of forty.

17.   Dysfunctional Sexual Process

Apart from the normal process of menopause there are a few female cases and also women in general terms have a low libido for sex in their daily lives. The orgasm process for female segment of society is a great difficulty for women class. This is just the opposite of their male counter partners. For male segment of society, orgasm is a normal process and an easily available process. These differences are the main reason that the women section of society usually remains unsatisfied during the sexual process and remain depressed and frustrated. When the female section of society takes a regular dose of the root then their anxiety level increases and thus the whole sexual process becomes pleasant for them and helps in alleviating the mood of both the partners equally. This is a great source of maintaining a great mental balance in the life of married couples and living a healthy and happy life.